LIST OF TOP 3 BATH AND BODY PRODUCTS

USER GUIDE FOR BATH AND BODY PRODUCTS

A.D RAMS

Contents

CHAPTER ONE

INTRODUCTION

Bath and body products are opulent delights that transform our everyday routines into indulgent and soothing moments when it comes to self-care and pampering. These products, which range from nourishing body creams to calming bath bombs, provide a sensory experience that revitalizes the body and uplifts the soul. This introduction will go over a carefully selected selection of the top three bath and body products that are well-known for their effectiveness, quality, and capacity to elevate regular self-care routines into remarkable blissful moments. These items will please your senses and leave you feeling renewed, energized, and completely pampered—whether you're wanting to relax after a long day or just treat yourself to a little pampering.

The Value of Taking Care of Oneself on a Daily Basis

It's simple to put work, family, and other commitments ahead of our personal needs in today's hectic environment where we frequently juggle several tasks and obligations. However, it is imperative that we include self-care into our daily routine in order to sustain our mental, emotional, and physical well-being. This is why taking care of oneself is crucial:

Stress reduction: Making time for self-care pursuits like walking, meditation, or physical activity can help lower stress levels and encourage relaxation. We can relax and recharge by partaking in things that make us happy and fulfilled, which eventually makes it easier for us to handle the rigors of everyday life.

Better Mental Health: Taking care of ourselves can make a big difference in our mental well-being. Journaling, being grateful, or going outside can all be effective ways to improve mood, lessen the signs of anxiety and depression, and improve mental health in general.

Improved Physical Health: Maintaining good physical health requires self-care habits including consistent exercise, a balanced diet, and enough sleep. Making these practices a priority not only helps us stay physically active but also boosts immunity, lowers the risk of chronic illnesses, and increases longevity.

Enhanced Productivity: Throughout the day, taking little breaks for self-care can really improve output and efficiency. We can work more productively and efficiently when we give ourselves time to relax and rejuvenate. This helps us return to work with more attention, energy, and motivation.

Improved interactions: We can be our best selves in our interactions with others when we put self-care first. Prioritizing our own needs allows us to be better able to assist, understand, and care for people around us, which promotes happier, healthier relationships.

Increased Resilience: Self-care serves as a protective barrier against life's obstacles and stressors. Regular self-nurturing helps us become more resilient, enhancing our capacity to overcome obstacles, overcome setbacks, and keep a positive attitude even under trying circumstances.

Incorporating self-care into our daily routine is crucial to preserving resilience, general health, and well-being. Making time for things that feed our mind, body, and soul a priority helps us handle stress better, maintain better mental and physical health, and create more pleasure and fulfillment in our lives. Recall that taking care of oneself is not selfish; rather, it is necessary for leading a healthy and contented life.

Exquisite Body Wash

Luxurious body scrubs are not only a sensory pleasure, but also a restorative experience that leaves your skin feeling smooth, soft, and glowing. The following justifies including an opulent body scrub in your self-care regimen:

Exfoliation: Dead skin cells are gently buffed away by a premium body scrub, exposing radiant, new skin underneath. Exfoliation makes the skin look younger and more radiant by encouraging cell turnover, clearing clogged pores, and improving texture and tone.

Moisture Balance: Nutritious oils and hydrating components are found in a lot of opulent body scrubs, which help restore moisture and seal in hydration. This lessens the appearance of dryness and roughness by softening and smoothing the skin as well as enhancing its suppleness and resilience.

Stress Reduction: Applying a rich body scrub to your skin can be a really soothing and healing experience. The calming aromas of aromatic plants or essential oils together with the mild exfoliation helps release stress, soothe the mind, and encourage a feeling of well-being and relaxation.

Benefits of Aromatherapy: Fragrant essential oils or botanical extracts are often included in opulent body washes. Choosing a body scrub with your favorite perfume will improve the sensory experience and brighten your mood, regardless of whether you love the exotic fragrance of jasmine, the invigorating aroma of citrus, or the peaceful scent of lavender.

Enhanced Circulation: Using a body scrub increases circulation through massage, which aids in lymphatic drainage, lowers fluid retention, and enhances the general health and vigor of your skin. An even skin tone and a healthy, glowing complexion can also be attributed to improved circulation.

Skin is Ready for Further Treatments: Using a high-end body scrub before using serums or moisturizers helps the ingredients go deeper and work better into the skin. A body scrub maximizes the advantages and increases the efficacy of other treatments by eliminating dead skin cells and unclogging pores.

Incorporating an opulent body scrub into your self-care regimen can provide numerous advantages for your skin, body, and mind. Whether you treat yourself to a lavish spa treatment or a monthly pampering session, a body scrub will leave you feeling renewed, invigorated, and completely pampered.

Nourishing body butter or lotion

A delightful treat for your skin, nourishing body butter or lotion provides moisture, nourishment, and a hint of decadence. For soft, supple, and healthy-looking skin, you must include a nourishing body lotion or body butter in your skincare routine for the following reasons:

Deep Moisturization: Body butters and lotions are made with emollient, rich ingredients like cocoa butter, shea butter, and organic oils like almond, jojoba, or coconut. Deep hydration and moisture replenishment are provided by these substances to dry, parched skin, leaving it feeling smooth, hydrated, and soft.

calming Relief: A nourishing body lotion or body butter can offer comfort and calming relief if you have dry, sensitive, or irritated skin. These products' creamy textures form a protective layer on the skin, reducing irritation brought on by dryness or environmental stresses as well as inflammation and redness.

Better Skin Texture: Using a body butter or lotion on a regular basis will help your skin look and feel better. These products' moisturizing ingredients smooth out uneven skin tone, soften rough spots, and generally encourage a healthier, more luminous complexion.

Long-Lasting Moisture: Body butters and thick body creams, as opposed to lighter lotions or moisturizers, give your skin long-lasting moisture and protection. Even in tough or dry environments, your skin will stay hydrated and comfortable because to their rich, occlusive formulations that seal in hydration and prevent moisture loss throughout the day.

Enhanced Fragrance: A lot of hydrating body butters and lotions are scented with aromatic essential oils or plant extracts to give your skincare regimen a pleasant aroma. Whether your preference is for fruity, floral, or herbal scents, picking a scented body butter or lotion can make you feel better about yourself and smell amazing all day.

Benefits Against Aging: Antioxidants, vitamins, and peptides are some of the chemicals included in some body lotions and body butters that help prevent aging-related symptoms like wrinkles, fine lines, and loss of suppleness. Over time, a more youthful and bright complexion is promoted by these nutritious nutrients that stimulate skin renewal, enhance collagen synthesis, and protect against environmental damage.

Maintaining healthy, moisturized, and beautiful skin requires including a nourishing body butter or lotion in your skincare routine. Choosing a product that matches your skin type and preferences will help maintain your skin looking and feeling its best every day, regardless of whether you prefer the rich texture of body butter or the lightweight feel of body lotion.

Bath salts or bombs with fragrance

Aromatic bath bombs or bath salts provide an opulent and decadent experience that turns a typical bath into a calming haven for the body, mind, and soul.

CHAPTER TWO

The following explains why adding fragrant bath bombs or bath salts to your self-care regimen is crucial for encouraging rest, renewal, and general wellbeing:

Stress Reduction: Fragrant essential oils, plant extracts, or aromatic herbs are blended into aromatic bath bombs or bath salts, which release their healing aromas into the water. By reducing stress, tension, and anxiety, inhaling these calming scents can encourage calmness and relaxation.

Muscle Relaxation: After a strenuous workout or a long day, bath bombs or bath salts with components like sea salt or Epsom salt (magnesium sulfate) can help ease discomfort and relax tired muscles. You can relax and let go of physical strain by taking use of the warm water and buoyancy of the bath.

Skin Nourishment: Skin-nourishing substances like coconut oil, shea butter, or vitamin E, which help moisturize, soften, and protect the skin, are frequently included in aromatic bath bombs or bath salts. Bath time becomes a luxurious pleasure for your skin because of these moisturizing components, which leave your skin feeling silky-smooth and supple.

Detoxification: Toxins, pollutants, and impurities can be drawn out of the skin by using bath bombs or bath salts mixed with detoxifying materials like seaweed, clay, or activated charcoal. This process helps the skin become cleaner and more detoxified. Your skin feels renewed, cleansed, and energized after this mild detox procedure.

Benefits of Aromatherapy: The benefits of aromatherapy, which can enhance mood, elevate spirits, and foster emotional well-being, are provided by aromatic bath bombs or bath salts. These products' healing smells can improve your bathing experience and encourage relaxation, whether you go for energizing scents like eucalyptus and peppermint or soothing ones like lavender and chamomile.

Better Sleep Quality: Before going to bed, take a warm bath with fragrant bath bombs or bath salts to help relax your body and mind and make it easier to fall asleep. The aromatherapy elements' peaceful scents when paired with the relaxing effects of the bath can encourage deeper, more comfortable sleep, leaving you feeling revived and renewed when you wake up.

Including fragrant bath bombs or bath salts in your self-care regimen has several advantages for your emotional, mental, and physical health. These products offer a lovely getaway that feeds the body, relaxes the mind, and restores the spirit whether you're wanting to unwind after a long day, ease aching muscles, or simply pamper yourself with a luxurious bath experience.

Comparative Analysis and Points to Remember

Aspects like components, advantages, smell, texture, and individual preferences should all be taken into account while contrasting and thinking about the top three bath and body products. Here is a comparison of each product and some things to think about:

Healthy Body Lotion:

Ingredients: Seek out body lotions that have natural oils like coconut, jojoba, or almond oil along with moisturizing ingredients like shea or cocoa butter. Steer clear of goods that include sulfates, parabens, artificial perfumes, and other potentially dangerous substances.

Benefits: Take into account the particular advantages provided by every body lotion, such as prolonged moisture retention, deep hydration, and calming comfort for dry or sensitive skin.

Scent: Pick a body lotion whose aroma pleases your senses and goes well with your taste preferences. Whether you like fruity, floral, or herbal smells, choose a product whose aroma elevates your spirits and makes the experience better all around.

Texture: Take note of the body lotion's consistency and texture. While some people prefer heavier creams or body butters for deeper hydration and nourishment, others might prefer lighter lotions that penetrate into the skin more rapidly.

Exquisite Body Wash:

Ingredients: Look for body scrubs that include nourishing oils and botanical extracts with natural exfoliants like sugar, salt, or crushed coffee. Products with harsh chemicals or microbeads that can harm skin should be avoided.

advantages: Take into account the moisturizing and exfoliating properties that every body scrub offers, including reduced stress levels, enhanced skin tone and texture, and aromatherapy advantages.

Scent: Pick a body scrub whose aroma pleases your senses and makes bathing more enjoyable. Choose a product that pampered and calms you, whether your preference is for exotic floral perfumes, relaxing lavender scents, or stimulating citrus scents.

Texture: Take into account the body scrub's texture and consistency. Fine-grain sugar scrubs are preferred by some people for a mild exfoliation, while salt scrubs are preferred by others for a more vigorous exfoliation. Select a texture based on your preferences and skin type.

Bath salts or bombs with fragrance:

Ingredients: Look for bath bombs or bath salts that are created with natural components, aromatic plant extracts, and essential oils. Steer clear of items that have harsh chemicals, artificial colors, or perfumes that can irritate your skin.

Benefits: Take into account how each bath bomb or bath salt promotes better sleep, detoxification, muscle relaxation, relaxation, and aromatherapy.

Scent: Pick bath bombs or bath salts that have aromas that soothe your senses and promote relaxation. Choose a product that boosts and encourages relaxation, whether your preference is for the stimulating citrus aroma, the calming lavender, or the refreshing eucalyptus.

Texture: Take into account the bath bombs' or the bath salts' dissolving qualities. While some people might favor bath salts that dissolve swiftly and evenly, releasing their aromatic scent and skin-nourishing substances, others might prefer bubbly bath bombs that release bubbles and color into the water.

It's critical to compare and take into account aspects like components, advantages, aroma, texture, and individual preferences while analyzing the top three bath and body products. Select skincare products based on your needs, interests, and values. Then, enjoy the exquisite sensation of indulging in opulent bath and body treatments.

Summary

When it comes to pampering and self-care, choosing the appropriate bath and body products may make your everyday routine feel opulent and decadent. It's clear from contrasting and weighing the top three bath and body products that each provides special advantages and indulgent experiences to improve your skincare routine and encourage rest, renewal, and general wellbeing.

These products take your self-care regimen to new levels of luxury and indulgence, whether you're nurturing your skin with a sumptuous body lotion, enjoying the blissful exfoliation of a body scrub, or submerging yourself in the scented ecstasy of bath bombs or bath salts.

These top three bath and body products prioritize luxurious textures, calming aromas, and high-quality ingredients to give nourishment, hydration, and relaxation. The result is skin that is luminous, smooth, and soft, and senses that are awakened and renewed.

In the end, adding these top three bath and body products to your daily regimen provides an opulent way to pamper yourself, nurture your skin, and savor the delights of self-care while also providing a lovely respite from the demands of everyday life. Use these excellent bath and body products to enhance your self-care regimen and give yourself the opulent experience you deserve.

THE END